I0449624

ESSENTIALLY FEMININE

ESSENTIAL OILS FOR EVERY WOMAN

Essentially Feminine
Essential Oils for Every Woman

Rebecca Samuels

Edition Notice

First printed 26 May 2015 by CreateSpace, LLC. as a
self-published work.

© Essentially Feminine, All Rights Reserved

ISBN: 978-1523964147

Typeface: Arial 11pt

Medical Disclaimer

The information provided is not intended to be a substitute for professional medical advice, diagnosis or treatment. Never disregard professional medical advice, or delay in seeking it, because of something you have read in this book. Never rely on information presented in this book in place of seeking professional medical advice.

I advocate being cleared by your medical professional before approaching a suitably qualified aromatherapist. Any reputable aromatherapist will insist on this, especially if you are undergoing fertility treatment, pregnant or breastfeeding.

Essentially Feminine is not responsible or liable for any advice, course of treatment, diagnosis or any other information, services or products that you obtain as a direct result of reading this book. You are encouraged to consult with your medical practitioner and suitable qualified aromatherapist with regard to any information contained within this book, and to take their advice.

Personal Disclaimer

I am a childbirth educator, Natural Womanhood advocate and a student aromatherapist, not a doctor.

The information I provide is based on my personal experience with and application of essential oils in conjunction with a qualified aromatherapist and the consent of medical professionals.

Anything recommended in this book should form the basis of discussion between yourself and your medical professional and/or qualified aromatherapist as essential oils are potent and their use carries risks.

Dedications

To my parents, Elizabeth and David, and my Uncle Zane, for encouraging my slavish adoration of books.

To my daughter, Neia, because when I was a little girl I always wanted to be in the dedications section of a book.

To my sister and best friend, Jadine, who is beyond compare- the Audrey to my Elizabeth, and the best co-conspirator a girl could ever wish for.

Contents

What Is Natural Womanhood?

Thank you for choosing to read *Essentially Feminine*. You have in your hands or your lap, the culmination of over ten years' experience and interaction with the properties of plants, which led to my work with essential oils and, ultimately, this book. Essentially Feminine is the combination of the therapeutic benefits, emotional and memory interaction and pleasant scents of aromatherapy with **Natural Womanhood**.

My life's work, **Natural Womanhood**, is based on two very simple tenets:
1. All women have the right to be supported through the milestones of life.
2. Nurturing with nature is the best path to follow.

In my work, studies and life experiences, I have learned that the most important person to nurture is yourself. We are all empty vessels, who can only give to others what we ourselves have- Stress and tension have no place in a family, whereas feelings of calm, peace and love lead us naturally by the hand to happier relationships of all kinds. I have chosen to teach women how to dive into their very souls, to pull up their fears by the roots and rebuild strong foundations where there was self-doubt and worse.

You, reading this book, have lived with your heart, which has taken you through the great changes of your life, knowing all the time there is more beneath the surface.

Please- Read on, and follow where the ripples and eddies of your soul tides lead...

*Walking with you through the labyrinth of womanhood,
in love and sacred trust.*

Rebecca Samuels
Essentially Feminine

Essential Oils and Aromatherapy

The value of essential oils and aromatherapy has been recognised for over 6,000 years, for their healing, cleansing, preservative and emotional properties, as well as the pleasure of their scents. Every civilisation in the world started with the burning of specific herbs and woods, believing the smoke would carry their prayers to the heavens; which led over the years to the highly specialised distillation of a plant's most minute benefits, and has, from its earliest days, used essential oils to enrich the physical, psychological and spiritual lives of its people.

This comes as no surprise when you learn there are 10 million cells in our nose, which transmit directly to the olfactory bulb. This is why memories around scent are often the longest-lasting and strongest we have. Think, for example, of lavender, or apple pie, or coffee!

The art and science of aromatherapy harnesses the many qualities of essential oils and the power of the senses of touch and smell. To use essential oils is, in fact, not to work with oils at all, but to work with highly concentrated plant extracts with powerful healing properties, which is why they should never be used directly on the skin. Carrier or base oils are bland, vegetable based oils used to "carry" the essential oils and dilute their potency. Essential oils should be stored away from heat, light and air, because they can evaporate or deteriorate.

Aromatherapy is at the same time a specific science, a deeply complex art and an ever-evolving challenge. To practice aromatherapy is to enjoy a knowledge of chemistry, botany and physiology, and to access thousands of years of personal use and experimentation. The direct link between our sense of smell and our memories and emotions, means scents can evoke an immediate and powerful reaction which has nothing to do with our usual thought processes and that defies rational analysis. Essential oils subtly affect mind, body and emotions in ways we're still studying and learning about. As essential oils cannot be patented, drugs companies will not fund research into them, but new research about essential oils is conducted all the time as we remember what our earliest forebears knew all along- Mother Nature takes care of her own!

Safety Warnings

Here are some basic safety warnings. Important information and warnings for each essential oil are listed with their profiles. Please note, I actively encourage you not to take this as a complete list, do be sure to conduct your own research as well:

- NEVER take essential oils internally!
- Dilute essential oil blends at a maximum of 3% (3 drops EO in 1 tsp carrier oil). If you are pregnant or breastfeeding, 1-2% is more advisable (1-2 drops EO in 1 tsp carrier oil).
- Take care in pregnancy with any oil- use only with professional advice. There is a lot of contention over which oils are safe or not during pregnancy, as it is obviously completely unethical to test potentially harmful substances on a pregnant woman, but the Natural Womanhood list has been carefully cross-referenced over many different reputable sources, and all contraindications are listed with the individual oils.
- Citrus oils can irritate the skin and react badly when exposed to sunlight.
- Alternative therapies are not a replacement for professional advice.
- ALWAYS get medical advice for serious or long term problems.
- If you get essential oil in your eyes, do NOT rinse with water. Carefully flush the eye clean with good quality vegetable oil- this will make

your vision slightly blurry, but that will pass. Once the blurriness has gone, then gently flush your eyes with very weak saline solution- a pinch of salt in a cup of water is a similar concentration to the salt level of tears.

- Please conduct a skin test with any new oils- use 1 drop in 1 tsp of carrier oil (sunflower oil is ideal) and leave for 24 hours. If any reaction happens, discontinue use. This is especially important in oils which may cause a reaction on sensitive skin, which are listed throughout this book.

It is almost impossible to create a conclusive list of "safe" oils. Professionals, even within the same organization, debate extensively over the use of certain oils. If you're ever unsure about an oil or its use, do all the research you can, and if you still can't make up your mind as to its safety- avoid it. But, by all means, do NOT be afraid of essential oils. Just use them with care and respect, and ideally in conjunction with a local, qualified aromatherapist, who will be able to prescribe you a list of essential oils you can use safely under their advice. While there is no conclusive list of "safe" oils, there is a very clearly outlined list of toxic oils which should be avoided.

How to Use Essential Oils

Bath oil
The essential oils recommended for the bath effect the body twofold, as they are inhaled in the steam and some also penetrate pores in the skin which open in the warm conditions. In order to add oils to the bath safely it is important to dilute them in cream or full fat milk, as vegetable leaves a dirty tidemark around the waterline of the bath. Add the blend to the bathwater, just as the bath reaches your desired depth, so the water disperses the additive, but before the essential oils can evaporate.

Diffusing
By far the safest way to use essential oils, and one of the most pleasant! Fill the reservoir half full with water, and add a few drops of your chosen essential oil. By lighting a candle under the reservoir, the blend is gently heated and the essential oils are diffused in the steam. The steam should diffuse slowly so the scent lasts a long time. A few drops of a skin-friendly essential oil in a bowl of warm water and left in a room serves the twofold role of humidifier and gentle skin tonic.

Flower Water for Skin Problems
Add your desired oils to a glass spray bottle filled with 100ml distilled water, put in a dark place and shake every day for a week before straining through a coffee filter. Store this mix in the fridge for a refreshing tonic for skin complaints. It should have therapeutic benefits for about a month if kept in the fridge.

Hand and Foot Baths

3-5 drops of essential oil in a tablespoon of milk swirled into a bowl of warm water makes a refreshing treat at the end of the day, or a pampering addition to a manicure or pedicure.

Handkerchief or Tissue

By dropping 3-5 drops of oil onto a handkerchief or tissue. you can inhale essential oils to relieve acute symptoms.

Hot or Cold Compresses

A pad soaked either in a bowl of warm or cool water with a touch of milk and a few drops of essential oil then gently bound to the affected area with bandages or medical tape makes a wonderful treatment. This is especially useful when warm, for period pain, or cool as a forehead compress in labour.

Inhalers

Take an empty nasal inhaler and roll the clean cotton insert in 15-18 drops of essential oil, then construct the inhaler for on-the-go aromatherapy treatment. Especially good for respiratory problems.

Massage

Almost everyone will benefit from a luxurious massage with a few drops of essential oil in a suitable base oil. The heady fragrance, beautifully beneficial oils and soothing strokes of a massage will rebalance your body and mind, leaving you perfectly relaxed and refreshed, ready to continue taking on the world.

A Note on Oils for Babies and Children

I would not recommend oils which are not safe for your precious bundles, that would be hugely remiss of me. All of the oils listed here are safe to use on young children at a 1% dilution, so 1 drop per teaspoon of carrier oil, but for children under 4 years of age I would recommend only diffusing oils for a short time (20-30 minutes) for your child to absorb their benefit indirectly, rather than applying them to the skin- Under the age of two, essential oils should be used under the careful guidance of a qualified aromatherapist, as a child's skin is much thinner than an adult's. Only use oils in places where young children are unlikely to be able to reach their mouths to the area, as essential oils cannot be ingested- the sole of the foot being a particularly popular area. Always seek medical advice if you even suspect your child may have ingested any essential oil.

Babies respond particularly well to massage, as they thrive on being touched, held and cuddled. Skin-to-skin contact with babies is essential to parent-baby bonding. However, any young child under the age of 4 should be massaged with pure base oil, sunflower oil is particularly gentle, as their skin is too sensitive to permit essential oil application. However, oils can be lightly diffused in minimal quantities for their indirect benefits:

Newborn infants: Chamomile, Geranium, Lavender, Mandarin and Rose can be diffused.
Babies 2-6 months old: Neroli can also be diffused.

Babies 6-12 months old: Eucalyptus, Peppermint and Tea Tree can also be diffused.

Babies 12+ months old: Frankincense, Marjoram, Rosemary, Sandalwood, Thyme and Ylang Ylang can also be diffused.

Babies 24+ months old: Chamomile, Lavender, Mandarin, Neroli, Rose, Palmarosa and Tea Tree- 1% dilution for application

Children 7-12 years: 1/4 dilution of adult strength.

A Note on Pregnancy

If you think you are pregnant, consult an aromatherapist immediately if you intend to begin or continue using essential oils. Pregnancy is a glorious time in our lives when many of us find ourselves yearning to rejoin a more harmonious relationship with nature, and aromatherapy is a very easy to learn, highly applicable skill to encourage this new development. By all means, take this book with you as a tool to launch a conversation with your aromatherapist, as they guide you through your precious nine months. They will be able to guide and teach you far better than this book ever could, as they have the advantage of a full intake interview, which may take a couple of hours to complete.

If you intend to use essential oils without the experience and knowledge of a qualified aromatherapist, then please read all you can about the oil you hope to use, and try to stick only to the recommendations of quality and trustworthy websites, such as http://www.aromaweb.com/.

This book provides you with a list of over 20 oils to research and consider in your aromatherapy usage during pregnancy. Please note, known emmenagogues (oils which bring on periods, and thus can hypothetically, in some cases, bring on miscarriage/spontaneous abortion) are listed in their profiles and should be avoided in pregnancy.

A Note on Diluting Oils

Diluting essential oils is, well, essential. Essential oils are too potent to apply straight to the skin, and thus they need a carrier oil to "carry" them onto the skin in a safe dilution. Suitable base oils include:

Sweet almond oil, probably the most versatile and useful.
Grapeseed oil, which is excellent for sensitive skins.
Sunflower oil, which is inexpensive, light and easily absorbed into the skin.
Olive oil, perfect for dry skins and often on hand in a kitchen.

As a luxurious addition, jojoba oil can be added at a maximum of 10% of a carrier oil blend. This is for a few reasons, not least because jojoba oil is an expensive addition to your aromatherapy practice! It does, however, last a very long time as it does not go rancid, and it is one of the closest approximations of human sebum, the natural skin oils we all have to some degree. This makes it easily absorbed, as well as a longer-lasting base oil.

If you are adding the oils to water, you may find the oil doesn't disperse properly- Substituting full fat milk or cream in place of the base oil, you will still have a carrier for the essential oils but they will not feel as greasy. An added benefit is the softening properties of the milk. If you are vegetarian or vegan, I would recommend using oil instead, but please do be careful as it may make the bathtub slippery as you get out.

Perfume Notes and Blending Aromatherapy Oils

Knowing a little about perfume notes, or the depth of scent and staying power of each essential oil, helps you create beautifully balanced oil blends whose therapeutic effects are magnified by each oil in the blend, each working together to enhance the blend. Essential oils fall into one of three notes:

Top notes: These are the lighter, fresh scents, which evaporate and fade quickly.
Heart notes: These are denser, more herbal and deeply floral scents, and this is the point at which you should decide if you like a perfume or not, as this is the longest lasting scent of a blend.
Base notes: These woody, earthy oils "fix" the scent, anchoring the blend and making it last longer.

Because of the interaction of the olfactory bulb with the limbic system, scents evoke our strongest and most powerful memories. It's time to get to know your essential oils. You don't have to have all the oils immediately to enjoy this section, but the more oils you have, the more practice you can get with blending. Start with your base note, add a couple of drops of the heart note then a drop of the top note. Personally, a blending ratio I can recommend is 1:3:2, from base to top note. For example:

1 drop Frankincense
3 drops Ylang Ylang

2 drops Lemon

Natural Womanhood- The Oils

The essential oils used for Natural Womanhood are carefully and lovingly selected to nurture all aspects of being a woman, both physically and emotionally, in a marriage of therapeutic and energetic aromatherapy. These oils and blends smell divine, are incredibly effective, and very much loved for their gentle interaction with the body. The essential oils covered in this book focus solely upon feminine health, and they have been meticulously chosen for their therapeutic, olfactory, energetic and synergistic effects on the body.

Please, once again, exercise caution when using any of the oils recommended in this book. Without the backing of a qualified aromatherapist to guide you and consider what works for your needs, this book is at best friendly advice.

I have used reasonable caution and many, many different sources of information to ascertain the level of safety of the listed oils for use in pregnancy, but they are only a guide. If you are pregnant, general advice suggests to use essential oils only after 12 weeks gestation, which is my advice, unless other limits are listed with individual oils. These profiles are not considered to be complete and is not guaranteed to be accurate. If you are not sure, do not use that oil.

I personally would not recommend use of essential oils on the skin in pregnancy, but diffusion should present no problems. If you intend to use essential oils in pregnancy, ask a professional aromatherapist's advice, but only ever use them at 1% dilution, or one drop in 1 tsp base oil. Please note, at the time of publishing, my research found no reports of problems in pregnancy or labour or of fetal health issues following essential oil use in pregnancy whilst using essential oils, but it's always better to be safe.

In the following pages, make a note of what memories each scent evokes for you. There are not right or wrong answers, there is only how you feel about a blend. What you bring to aromatherapy in personal memory and experience of scents, is just as important as the technical knowledge you learn about blending.

For ease, the oils are listed in alphabetical order.

Bergamot

Bergamot's best qualities are pain reducing, antidepressant, antiseptic, calming, invigorating and healing. Bergamot is invaluable for psychological and emotional states such as insomnia, anxiety, depression, emotional imbalance, fear and tension, and is best used at the start of the day. Burn in a diffuser to lift the atmosphere and regain self-confidence. It is also a fantastic healing oil to use for cystitis and cramps. Bergamot is phototoxic, so do not use it on skin exposed to sunlight. Don't use Bergamot on your skin in pregnancy, but you can diffuse it to reap its benefits.

It blends well with Chamomile, Cypress, Geranium, Jasmine, Lavender, Lemon, Mandarin, Neroli, Rose, Sandalwood, Vetiver and Ylang Ylang. Bergamot is a top note.

Virginia Cedarwood

Cedarwood is thought to be one of the earliest known essential oils, and Virginia Cedarwood is considered safer than Atlas Cedarwood. Its best qualities are its antiseptic, cramp-alleviating and invigorating effects. It's fantastic for calming, relaxation and soothing both mind and body, and is uplifting when treating lack of confidence or fearfulness. Use Cedarwood in meditations to boost courage and inner resolve, and reduce fear- It is as bolstering as it is comforting and calming. Both men and women enjoy its scent, and its properties make it ideal to diffuse or inhale in the labour room. Don't use Cedarwood oil on your skin in pregnancy, but you can diffuse it to reap its benefits. If you are not pregnant and wish to use it on your skin, use it at a 1% dilution under the advice of an aromatherapist, but be aware Cedarwood can cause skin irritation, so should be used for a maximum of two concurrent weeks and only after a skin test.

It blends well with Bergamot, Chamomile, Clary Sage, Cypress, Eucalyptus, Jasmine, Lavender, Neroli, Petitgrain, Rosemary, Sandalwood, Vetiver and Ylang Ylang. Cedarwood is a base note.

German Chamomile

German Chamomile numbs pain and helps scar tissue to form and wounds to heal. It relieves muscle aches, toothache and inflammation. Chamomile oil is relaxing and helps deaden the pain of cramps, which makes it fantastic for indigestion and other digestive problems. In pregnancy, the scent of Chamomile can help reduce morning sickness. Its pronounced effect on the nervous system and the mind makes Chamomile useful for meditations where there is a feeling of being hysterical or out of control. It also relieves anxiety, tension headaches, stress, insomnia and PMT. A blend of Chamomile and Clary Sage is particularly good for period pains and irritability.

Chamomile is indispensable for children even as very young babies, as its gentle soothing and numbing qualities make it ideal for every complaint from colic, immunisation sites and teething time.

Chamomile blends well with Bergamot, Clary Sage, Frankincense, Geranium, Jasmine, Lavender, Lemon, Mandarin, Marjoram, Neroli, Patchouli, Rose, Rosemary, Tea Tree and Ylang Ylang. Chamomile is a top note.

Clary Sage

Clary Sage is a powerful antiseptic renowned for relieving pain and assisting with healing. It's also a fantastic antidepressant, which induces a sense of wellbeing and gives a euphoric uplift to the brain; be careful how much you use, however, as it can leave you feeling very intoxicated! Great in a relaxing bath. Clary Sage helps to lift the spirits, be receptive to outside influences, which is useful for labour, and is a powerful sedative and nervous tonic. Clary Sage is helpful for painful periods and menopausal symptoms, and is especially appropriate for meditations about first periods and the approach of the menopause.

Not recommended for use if you suffer with high blood pressure or epilepsy. If pregnant, avoid until you are in labour- it is well known to induce periods. In labour, it makes a highly effective painkiller.

It blends well with Bergamot, Cedarwood, Chamomile, Cypress, Frankincense, Jasmine, Lavender, Lemon, Mandarin, Patchouli, Petitgrain, Rose, Sandalwood and Tea Tree. Clary Sage is a heart note.

Cypress

Cypress is calming and antiseptic. With a scent similar to pine needles, Cypress is fantastic when added to a bath to help relieve fluid retention as it is a powerful astringent, used to dry up excess fluid. Cypress is especially good for varicose veins, hemorrhoids, swollen ankles and tired aching feet and legs. It is uplifting in cases of sadness and depression,and can help to soothe anger. Psychologically, it is useful to meditate with when the mind is overactive. Don't use Cypress on your skin in early pregnancy, but you can diffuse it to reap its benefits. If you wish to use it on your skin, use it at a 1% dilution under the advice of an aromatherapist, after 20 weeks.

Blends well with Cedarwood, Chamomile, Clary Sage, Ginger, Lavender, Lemon, Mandarin and Ylang Ylang. Cypress is a heart note.

Eucalyptus

Eucalyptus is a very effective antiseptic, which is also good for aches, pains and general healing, Excellent for breathing difficulties, Eucalyptus is a fantastic essential oil to use if you suffer with asthma. Well diluted in a carrier oil, Eucalyptus can be applied to the forehead to help relieve a hot, tense headache linked with tiredness. Eucalyptus dispels fatigue, clears the mind and helps you to face the day ahead. The use of Eucalyptus is not recommended for use if you take homeopathic remedies. Eucalyptus can cause skin irritation, so should be used for a maximum of two concurrent weeks. Eucalyptus is a fantastic oil to use for the whole family in homemade head-lice repelling treatments.

Blends well with Cedarwood, Chamomile, Cypress, Geranium, Ginger, Lavender, Lemon, Marjoram, Peppermint, Rosemary and Thyme. Eucalyptus is a top note.

Frankincense

Frankincense is one of the oldest essential oils used in meditation and spiritual practice, with the added benefit of being a general skin tonic. It has the effect of slowing and deepening our breathing, which lends itself to feeling calm and centred when we are anxious, nervous or stressed. It naturally works to relax the user and lower blood pressure. Frankincense aids sleep, good in the bath to treat stress. As well as being anti-inflammatory and antiseptic, Frankincense is great for healing the skin.

Blends well with Bergamot, Cypress, Geranium, Lavender, Lemon, Mandarin, Neroli, Patchouli, Rose, Sandalwood, Vetiver and Ylang Ylang. Frankincense is a base note.

Geranium

Geranium is well known as "The Womens' Oil"! Its painkilling, antidepressant, antiseptic and healing properties are well-documented, and emotionally Geranium lends itself as a great balancing oil, indicated when you feel unbalanced, indecisive or rigid and stuck. It is useful when meditating on life changes when we need to find harmony and balance in our lives, such as first periods, pregnancy and the onset of the menopause, easing the flow of these transitions. It works marvellously well as a tonic for the adrenal glands, balancing the hormones naturally, which means it is indispensable for "women's troubles" such as irregular or painful periods, PMS and menopausal changes, used to help with fluid retention, aching legs and poor circulation. As such, don't use Geranium in pregnancy.

Relaxing and refreshing, Geranium works wonders on nervous tension and exhaustion, and can combine a blend to make a more harmonious scent. It is, however, a strong scent, so not much is needed or you run the risk of overpowering your blend.

Blends well with Bergamot, Chamomile, Clary Sage, Cypress, Ginger, Jasmine, Lemon, Mandarin, Neroli, Patchouli, Peppermint, Rose, Rosemary, Sandalwood and Ylang Ylang. Geranium is a heart note.

Ginger

Ginger oil is known for its warm and comforting nature. It is a balancing oil and counteracts muscular aches and pains.

Ginger is an emotional tonic, excellent for meditations to alleviate nervous exhaustion, and helps build courage to inspire action. Its zingy fragrance cuts through nausea and nerves, and when blended with neroli encourages you to "feel the fear but do it anyway", making it indispensable in labour. Ginger oil is very strong, so it is best diffused for its benefits. If you wish to use it physically, try making ginger tea with fresh, stewed ginger, rather than using the essential oil.

Blends well with Bergamot, Cedarwood, Eucalyptus, Frankincense, Geranium, Jasmine, Lemon, Mandarin, Neroli, Patchouli, Rose, Sandalwood, Vetiver and Ylang Ylang. Ginger is both a heart and a base note, depending on the quality of the oil and the oils it is blended with, but for the purposes of this book we will consider it a heart note.

Jasmine

Jasmine is the undisputed king of the essential oils, potent and expensive. It has a powerful relaxing, euphoric effect, and can lift the mood when there is depression and general listlessness. It is both a sedative and an antidepressant, but it is not an oil for doing nothing! Use Jasmine in meditations to clear emotional blocks, as it acts as a nervous tonic. The sense of mystery in the fragrance helps you to allow life to happen freely, without having to control events. It is very much a go-with-what-feels-natural oil. Only a little Jasmine oil is needed in a blend, which makes a usually cost-prohibitive oil very economical!

Avoid Jasmine in pregnancy, but it's powerfully helpful in small quantities when diffused in labour. It's also reputed to increase milk production postpartum, so can be diffused or inhaled to gain its benefits. Please, do not apply anything to your breasts while breastfeeding to increase milk production, but review my notes on Breastfeeding under The Journey of Pregnancy.

Blends well with Bergamot, Clary Sage, Ginger, Lemon, Mandarin, Neroli, Patchouli, Petitgrain, Rose, Sandalwood and Ylang Ylang. Jasmine is a heart note.

Lavender

Lavender is the best-known and most widely used of all essential oils. It is an unbelievably adaptable and effective oil- Antiseptic, antidepressant, as well as being an effective relief for pain, stress and insomnia. Lavender can stimulate appetite and cell renewal, help heal minor wounds and burns, relieve muscular aches and pains, fluid retention, digestive problems and headaches.

Makes a soothing bath to promote restful sleep, as it is sedative in larger doses. Lavender is useful in meditations to focus the mind if it swings from one thing to another. It also clears the head and is useful for indecisiveness. It is also good for clearing emotional pain felt in the heart.

Blends well with Bergamot, Cedarwood, Chamomile, Clary Sage, Cypress, Eucalyptus, Geranium, Lemon, Mandarin, Marjoram, Patchouli, Peppermint, Rose, Rosemary, Tea Tree, Thyme and Vetiver. Lavender is both a top and a heart note, but for the purposes of this book, we will consider it a top note.

Lemon

The most cleansing and antiseptic of the citrus oils, Lemon oil is fresh, bright and undeniably citrusy. Lemon is most effective in preventing emotional outbursts, and can refresh and clarify thoughts, preventing feelings of bitterness or anger about life's injustices. It's particularly useful in pregnancy as an energising and uplifting oil to help with morning sickness and varicose veins, and in childbirth for homebirth-to-hospital transfers. Lemon has been proven to help aid concentration by clearing the mind and aiding the decision-making process. It is indispensable for meditations to clear a foggy and confused mind, to help ease psychological trauma and to purify and cleanse the mind.

Lemon oil is phototoxic, so do not use it on skin exposed to sunlight. It can cause skin irritation.

Blends well with Chamomile, Eucalyptus, Frankincense, Geranium, Lavender, Neroli, Rose, Sandalwood and Ylang Ylang. Lemon is a top note.

Mandarin

Mandarin is also known as "the children's oil" for it's gentle, calming but effective action. It acts effortlessly to soothe heartburn and nausea and calm fluid retention and swollen legs. A wonderfully cheerful and uplifting oil, acting as an emotional tonic, it is excellent in synergy with Bergamot, as it amplifies the properties of the cheerful, uplifting blend. Mandarin is mildly hypnotic in meditative blends, and soothes a racing mind. Use it to clear the mind of old thoughts and issues, to literally blow away the cobwebs. It has a strengthening effect on the nerves.

Mandarin is phototoxic, so do not use it on skin exposed to sunlight.

Blends well with Chamomile, Clary Sage, Frankincense, Geranium, Jasmine, Lemon, Neroli, Patchouli, Petitgrain, Rose, Sandalwood and Ylang Ylang. Mandarin is a top note.

Marjoram

Marjoram helps with pain on all levels, thought especially muscular complaints caused by swelling and is a great nurturer and comforter. Its action is slightly numbing. This oil has a calming and warming effect, and is good for women who might also suffer from headaches, migraines or insomnia. In ancient times, marjoram was chewed to deaden toothache, so a drop in a teaspoon of carrier oil massaged under the temples and under the jawline to calm inflamed nerves will help immensely. As well as helping soothe all kinds of pain, Marjoram works fantastically well as an antiseptic, healing oil and a general tonic. Due to its powerful painkilling effects, Marjoram is only recommended in labour if pregnant.

Blends well with Bergamot, Cedarwood, Chamomile, Cypress, Eucalyptus, Lavender, Lemon, Mandarin, Peppermint, Rosemary, Tea Tree and Thyme. Marjoram is a heart note.

Neroli

Neroli is an amazingly calming oil, gentle but powerful, and unsurpassed for dealing with shock, hysteria and nervous tension. It has a powerful psychological effect, reaching deep into the psyche to bring calm and stability. An excellent sedative and antidepressant, Neroli slows and calms the mind, allowing thoughts to clear and settle and strengthening the nerves. Neroli brings tranquillity, creating a feeling of peace and is useful during times of anxiety, panic, hysteria, shock or fear. Physically, Neroli acts to relieve tension, headaches, insomnia and other stress-related conditions, and upset stomachs. Only a little Neroli is needed in a blend, to prevent it overpowering the synergy.

Blends well with Chamomile, Clary Sage, Frankincense, Geranium, Ginger, Jasmine, Lavender, Lemon, Mandarin, Petitgrain, Rose, Sandalwood and Ylang Ylang. Neroli is a heart note.

Patchouli

Patchouli has a scent you either love or loathe, and many people raised in the 1960s have strong memories surrounding its scent. Soothing and grounding, Patchouli can "earth" our energy, rooting us safely within ourselves if we are anxious or tense. A little goes a long way in blends, and the scent lingers well. Patchouli is a very useful oil, as it is stimulating in small doses and sedative in larger doses. It is good to relax aching feet when used in the bath, or to reduce morning sickness if diffused in an oil burner. As well as being an excellent antidepressant and tonic, Patchouli helps dispel anxiety, being gently stimulating to emotions, and easing confusion, indecision and apathy.

Blends well with Bergamot, Cedarwood, Chamomile, Clary Sage, Frankincense, Geranium, Ginger, Jasmine, Lavender, Mandarin, Neroli, Rose, Sandalwood and Vetiver. Patchouli is a base note.

Peppermint

Peppermint's zingy and fresh scent is powerfully uplifting, stimulating and enhances alertness. Its painkilling and cramp-relieving qualities make it very useful for rubbing onto the temples to relieve tension headaches, diluted in a teaspoon of carrier oil. In stronger dilutions, Peppermint is a calming and relaxing oil. Considered safe after 16 weeks gestation when pregnant. Not recommended for use if you take homeopathic remedies. Can cause skin irritation.

Blends well with Eucalyptus, Geranium, Lavender, Lemon, Marjoram, Rosemary and Tea Tree. Peppermint is a top note.

Petitgrain

Petitgrain is antiseptic and relaxes the body. It is particularly useful for fatigue, because it refreshes and stimulates the mind and is generally relaxing and balancing, indispensable in dealing with pre and postnatal depression. Used in a calming bath blend, Petitgrain acts well after birth to help repair the body and cope with the demands faced by new mothers.

Blends well with Bergamot, Cedarwood, Clary Sage, Cypress, Eucalyptus, Frankincense, Geranium, Jasmine, Lavender, Lemon, Mandarin, Marjoram, Neroli, Rose, Rosemary, Sandalwood and Ylang Ylang. Petitgrain is a top note.

Rose

Rose is the queen of essential oils to Jasmine's king. Roses symbolise life, death and rebirth, and the value of Rose oil cannot be overestimated. Rose strengthens and tones the reproductive organs in both sexes, treating menstrual disorders, and is excellent for use around the menopause, as it's fantastic for mature skin. Rose is good for sedating, calming and as an effective anti-inflammatory, soothes muscular and nervous tension.

It has deep psychological benefits, balancing and comforting. It reduces fear and reveals wisdom, creating an easier transition at times of immense emotional change. Rose is a powerful antidepressant, it cuts through anxiety, stress, depression and low self confidence to lift the spirits while acknowledging and soothing pain, anxiety, stress and sadness.

Rose is widely considered safe for use in pregnancy after 16 weeks gestation.

Blends well with Bergamot, Chamomile, Clary Sage, Frankincense, Geranium, Ginger, Jasmine, Lavender, Lemon, Mandarin, Neroli, Patchouli, Petitgrain, Sandalwood and Ylang Ylang. Rose is a heart note.

Rosemary

Rosemary has been used as incense since ancient times, and is one of the strongest mental stimulant oils there are. It works fantastically well for uncovering deeply rooted experiences, exposing them and clearing them. Combined with calming Neroli, stimulating Rosemary strengthens the mind ahead of trials and tribulations.

Balancing and uplifting on the emotions, Rosemary eases muscle and mental fatigue and is good for clearing the mind. This stimulating oil has been used for centuries to help relieve nervous exhaustion, tension headaches and migraines. It is an effective remedy for fluid retention, and works well to reduce pain.

Rosemary is not recommended for use if you suffer with high blood pressure or epilepsy, and it isn't recommended for use in pregnancy before 16 weeks gestation.

Blends well with Bergamot, Cedarwood, Clary Sage, Eucalyptus, Frankincense, Geranium, Lavender, Lemon, Mandarin, Marjoram, Peppermint, Petitgrain and Tea Tree. Rosemary is a heart note.

Sandalwood

Probably the oldest perfume in history, sandalwood has been used for 4,000 years. It has a heavy scent and is popular with both sexes. It has a relaxing, anti-depressant effect on the nervous system, as it restores equilibrium and is ideally used in a diffuser during labour to calm both parents. It is useful when there is a need to slow down and relax, so is useful for late pregnancy when you need all the relaxation you can get before the baby comes. As well as its calming emotional effects, Sandalwood is antiseptic, and can reduce fluid retention, cystitis and insomnia. It's gentle but thoroughly effective against viral infections.

Blends well with Bergamot, Chamomile, Clary Sage, Geranium, Frankincense, Jasmine, Lavender, Lemon, Mandarin, Neroli, Patchouli, Rose, Vetiver and Ylang Ylang. Sandalwood is a base note.

Tea Tree

Tea tree oil is naturally phenomenally effective at fighting many different microorganisms, from fungus to microbes. A very antiseptic oil, especially germicidal and antiviral, it is also a powerful immune stimulant, increasing the body's ability to respond to these organisms. This makes it amazing for acute symptoms of viral and bacterial infections during pregnancy, though especially against thrush and viral infections, when strong allopathic medications are ill-advised. Diffuse with lemon to create a fresh, invigorating scent whilst disinfecting a space.

Blends well with Bergamot, Chamomile, Clary Sage, Eucalyptus, Geranium, Lavender, Lemon, Marjoram, Peppermint, Rosemary, Thyme and Ylang Ylang. Tea Tree is a heart note.

Thyme

Thyme oil is strongly painkilling and cramp-alleviating, working effectively as an antibacterial and antiseptic oil. Thyme has a strongly beneficial effect on the circulatory system, essential in pregnancy what with the added strain the heart is put under, and on the digestive system, relieving excess gas. Thyme is also excellent to help stimulate healing, and relaxes sore aching muscles- Historically, feet and legs would be massaged with oil scented with Thyme. The scent is fresh and smells like a lazy summer evening when blended with Patchouli and Lemon. It also helps aid the memory and stimulates activity.

Blends well with Bergamot, Clary Sage, Cypress, Eucalyptus, Geranium, Lavender, Lemon, Marjoram, Rosemary and Tea Tree. Thyme is a heart note.

Vetiver

Vetiver is painkilling, invigorating in small doses and calming in large doses, antibacterial, antiseptic and stimulates healing, particularly of stretch marks. Vetiver has the added benefit of acting as a gentle aphrodisiac, so can inspire intimate moments between soon-to-be new parents, and can benefit those who suffer with insomnia. However, Vetiver is a strong but sweet scent, and quite divisive- You genuinely either love or hate it.

Blends well with Bergamot, Cedarwood, Clary Sage, Geranium, Ginger, Jasmine, Lavender, Lemon, Mandarin, Patchouli, Rose, Sandalwood and Ylang Ylang. Vetiver is a base note.

Ylang Ylang

Ylang Ylang means "Flower of flowers", and is used to induce a sense of euphoria. It has been proven to stimulate the release of endorphins in the brain, and as such it has a powerful effect on the nervous system. It has a potent effect on the body, and has a pleasant, though intense fragrance. Ylang Ylang has a sedative yet antidepressant action. It acts as a restorative for many symptoms of excessive tension, such as insomnia, panic attacks, fear, anxiety and depression, as well as lowering blood pressure. A good addition to baths and massage blends, especially postpartum as it has a gently antiseptic effect and helps promote healing.

Combined with Clary Sage, it creates a potent blend to help with the early stages of labour, by relieving the pain of contractions in two ways- Clary Sage is analgesic, and the euphoric state Ylang Ylang can induce releases endorphins and serotonin to help the body manage the pain more effectively.

Blends well with Bergamot, Chamomile, Clary Sage, Eucalyptus, Ginger, Jasmine, Lemon, Mandarin, Neroli, Patchouli, Petitgrain, Rose, Sandalwood and Vetiver. Ylang Ylang is both a heart and a base note, but for the purposes of this book we will consider it a heart note.

The Blends

A blend of essential oils in which the whole is greater
than the sum of its parts is known as a synergy. The
knowledge, awareness and listening skills required to
create synergies is quite complex. The creation of
blends in which the balance of essential oils within the
synergy is both therapeutically useful and aesthetically
pleasing is an art that is mastered only through study,
continual practice and personal experience. I am
fortunate enough to be able to whip synergistic blends
up with holistic effects for both myself and others
through much trial, error and practice, but now I almost
don't see the oils, I see a list of their effects and
harmonies. This is a skill I have honed over a long, long
period of study and experience, but I pass the benefit of
my experience on to you in the next two chapters.

All the essential oil blends are tried and tested, and
have benefited me or a friend personally. I leave the
actual choice of oils up to you in "Blends by Mood", as
everyone's emotional response to their scents is
different, and your tastes will probably be different to
mine, but "Product Blends" contains actual recipes I
love, use and heartily recommend.

Blends by Mood

A selection of essential oil blends by desired effect is given here, to be used as a guide. Choose three or four oils from each list to create your own blends:

Relaxing
Bergamot, Chamomile, Clary Sage, Frankincense, Jasmine, Lavender, Lemon, Mandarin, Marjoram, Neroli, Patchouli, Peppermint, Petitgrain, Rose, Sandalwood, Vetiver, Ylang Ylang

Uplifting
Cypress, Eucalyptus, Ginger, Jasmine, Lemon, Peppermint, Rosemary, Tea Tree, Thyme

For Stiff Muscles
Clary Sage, Eucalyptus, Geranium, Ginger, Jasmine, Lavender, Lemon, Mandarin, Marjoram, Peppermint, Rosemary, Vetiver

To Reconnect with your Partner
Cedarwood, Jasmine, Mandarin, Patchouli, Rose, Sandalwood, Vetiver, Ylang Ylang and any other oils you and your partner both find appealing.

Energising
Bergamot, Eucalyptus, Frankincense, Ginger, Lemon, Peppermint, Petitgrain, Rosemary, Tea Tree, Ylang Ylang

Balancing

Cedarwood, Cypress, Geranium

Product Blends

Hand Sanitiser

This blend is bought by chefs to be used in professional kitchens- The aloe vera is excellent for healing cuts and bruises, the witch hazel cools and tingles as it works hard at disinfecting your hands and the tea tree and lavender oils are antibacterial, antiseptic and antimicrobial as well as being strongly healing. You can use this as a hand sanitiser for everything from labour to nappy changing. You can even wipe down baby changing facilities with it, on a wad of paper towel! Don't worry about making so much at once, it's really versatile and lasts for at least six months, just shake it up before each use.

> 100 ml glass pump or flip cap bottle
> 75 ml pure aloe vera gel
> 25 ml witch hazel
> 24 drops tea tree
> 36 drops lavender

Abdominal Cramp Blend

This is best whipped up on the spot, or carried in a small bottle for a maximum of a week. If you need more, remember the 3% rule and multiply up accordingly. 5 ml is more than enough oil to perform a gentle abdominal massage.

For period pain
> 2 drops Lavender
> 1 drop Clary Sage

5 ml carrier oil

For labour contractions (5% is a strong painkilling blend)
     3 drops Lavender
     2 drops Clary Sage
     5 ml carrier oil

Homemade Head-Louse Repellent

This blend was used by my mother before me, when myself and my brother were young. Despite multiple outbreaks of head-lice at school, neither of us was ever infested. This blend was added to whole bottles of cheap conditioner and thoroughly mixed through, and applied to hair in a thick layer in order to trap and comb out the lice and eggs. It is possible to use it blended with diluted witch hazel in a spray bottle, too. This blend is best added to at least 500ml of conditioner.

Conditioner blend
     500 ml cheap conditioner
     50 drops Tea Tree
     25 drops Lavender
     10 drops Eucalyptus
     10 drops Rosemary
     5 drops Lemon

The quantities should be halved for the spray bottle, and 150 ml witch hazel should be diluted with 100 ml cooled distilled water. Store this blend in a glass bottle, as plastic bottles may be affected by the ingredients.

Witch Hazel blend
   150 ml Witch Hazel
   100 ml distilled water
   25 drops Tea Tree
   12 drops Lavender
   5 drops Eucalyptus
   5 drops Rosemary
   2 drops Lemon

Health Concerns

Under this section, you will find feminine complaints and the Natural Womanhood oils I have carefully and lovingly selected for their beneficial natures.

Many of the essential oils under Menstrual Problems are known to induce periods, so avoid them in pregnancy.

Menstrual Problems

Oh, it's good to be a woman! From the first spots of brown-red blood and dull ache in our bellies, to the joys and wisdom of menopause, we may on occasion face any one of a wealth of problems as menstruating women.

The major cause of most problems facing most menstruating women is anaemia, or iron deficiency- The average woman loses 15mg iron over the course of her monthly period, and can lose up to 500mg in pregnancy! An iron rich diet is essential for healthy, and therefore more comfortable, periods, so be sure to ask your doctor for a blood test to check for anaemia and keep your iron levels up!

The essential oils in this list are all fabulous when used traditionally, to assist with menstrual problems on many levels.

Amenorrhea (lack of periods)
How to use: Bath, inhalation, massage, vaporisation.
Clary Sage, Marjoram, Rose

Cystitis
How to use: Bath, compress, douche
Bergamot, Cedarwood, Chamomile, Eucalyptus, Frankincense, Lavender, Sandalwood, Tea Tree, Thyme

Dysmenorrhea (painful periods)
How to use: Bath, compress, inhalation, massage,

vaporisation.
Chamomile, Clary Sage, Frankincense, Jasmine, Lavender, Marjoram, Rose, Rosemary

Itching
How to use: 9 drops in a tablespoon of milk, swirled in a shallow bath
Bergamot, Cedarwood, Lavender, Tea Tree

Menopausal Problems
How to use: Bath, inhalation, massage, vaporisation.
Chamomile, Cypress, Geranium, Jasmine, Rose

Menorrhagia (heavy periods)
How to use: Bath, inhalation, massage, vaporisation.
Chamomile, Cypress, Rose

PMS
How to use: Bath, inhalation, massage, vaporisation.
Bergamot, Chamomile, Geranium, Lavender, Marjoram, Neroli, Rosemary

Thrush
How to use: As for Itching
Bergamot, Geranium, Tea Tree

Urethritis
How to use: As for Itching
Bergamot, Tea Tree

The Journey of Pregnancy: Pregnancy, Labour, Childbirth and Postpartum Problems

Pregnancy is, without a doubt, a magical time. Your senses become those of a superheroine, your personal insights are enhanced and your body proves itself to be an amazing creation- As we create new life, our minds and emotions change and morph at their slightest uncontrollable whim, our bodies change and our uteri expand an amazing 1000 times their usual capacity to accommodate our babies and hormones surge and rage within us. At the end of labour pains more intense than the pain we as humans consider survivable, spurred gently on by spiking oxytocin levels, we are repaid endlessly with a beautiful new baby who has grown from a simple fusing of two cells to the perfect bundle of new life we cradle to our bountiful breasts, flooded with milk which constantly adapt to the needs, hungers and requirements of our babies, transferring antibodies to guard against infections and the perfect balance of nutrients to ensure solid, swift weight gain for our inquisitive little angels.

Superwoman, indeed!

Aches and Pains
How to use: Bath, compress, massage
Chamomile, Clary Sage (labour), Eucalyptus, Lavender, Marjoram (labour), Peppermint, Rosemary, Thyme, Vetiver

Anxiety
How to use: Bath, massage, vaporisation
Bergamot, Frankincense, Jasmine (labour), Lavender, Neroli, Ylang Ylang

Breastfeeding
What to do: Do not wash breasts with strongly scented products, consider latching on techniques, seek a lactation consultant, feed and/or express frequently. Please do not consider me remiss in not mentioning any oils to apply to the skin in order to stimulate milk production, but there is a good reason for this. It isn't recommended to put anything on the breasts or nipples while breastfeeding. The strong smells would mask the natural odour of your postnatal breasts and confuse the baby, as nipples smell like amniotic fluid so the baby is attracted by the familiar smell after birth. During regular breastfeeding, the nipples produce their own cleaning agents, which is why you don't have to wash them with more than water while breastfeeding. I have not listed oils to help with pain, as if you've got a good latch going you should never feel actual pain. If you've already got sore nipples, see a lactation consultant to get help with your technique- Most breastfeeding discomforts disappear with a correct latch and frequent feeds. I can

recommend a lactation tea to help:

1/3 fenugreek seeds
2/3 fennel seeds

Mix in a jar to store, and steep two teaspoons in hot water for 5-7 minutes before drinking. Sweeten with organic honey or agave nectar to taste, and drink 3-4 cups daily.

How to use: Diffusion, inhalation, vaporisation
Jasmine

Depression
How to use: Bath, massage, vaporisation
Bergamot, Clary Sage (postpartum), Jasmine (postpartum), Lavender, Neroli, Rose, Sandalwood, Vetiver, Ylang Ylang

Headache
How to use: Compress, massage, vaporisation
Chamomile, Clary Sage (postpartum), Eucalyptus, Lavender, Marjoram, Peppermint, Rose, Rosemary, Thyme

Hemorrhoids and Piles
How to use: Bath, compress, skin oil
Cypress, Geranium

Indigestion
How to use: Massage

Chamomile, Clary Sage (postpartum), Ginger, Lavender, Mandarin, Marjoram (postpartum), Neroli, Peppermint, Petitgrain, Rosemary, Thyme

Insomnia
How to use: Bath, massage, vaporisation
Chamomile, Lavender, Mandarin, Marjoram (postpartum), Neroli, Petitgrain, Rose, Sandalwood, Thyme

Labour Pain, Childbirth Aid
How to use: Bath, Compress, Massage
Clary Sage (labour), Jasmine (labour), Lavender, Peppermint, Rose

Muscular Cramp
How to use: Bath, compress, massage
Clary Sage (labour), Cypress, Ginger, Jasmine (labour), Lavender, Marjoram (labour), Neroli, Peppermint, Rosemary, Thyme, Vetiver

Nausea and Vomiting
How to use: Massage, vaporisation
Chamomile, Ginger, Lavender, Peppermint, Rose, Sandalwood

Nervous Exhaustion and Fatigue
How to use: Bath, massage, vaporisation
Bergamot, Cedarwood, Chamomile, Clary Sage (labour), Cypress, Frankincense, Jasmine (labour), Lavender, Mandarin, Marjoram (labour), Neroli,

Patchouli, Peppermint, Petitgrain, Rose, Rosemary,
Sandalwood, Thyme, Vetiver, Ylang Ylang

Poor Circulation
How to use: Bath, massage,
Cypress, Eucalyptus, Geranium, Ginger, Lemon, Neroli,
Rose, Rosemary, Thyme

Scars and Stretch Marks
How to use: Massage, skin oil
Frankincense, Lavender, Mandarin, Neroli, Patchouli,
Sandalwood

Shock
How to use: Bath, massage, vaporisation
Lavender, Neroli

Slack Tissue
How to use: Bath, massage, skin oil
Geranium, Mandarin, Marjoram (postpartum), Neroli,
Petitgrain, Rosemary

Water Retention
How to use: Bath, massage
Cypress, Geranium, Mandarin, Rosemary

Wounds
How to use: Bath, compress, skin oil
Bergamot, Chamomile, Clary Sage (postpartum),
Cypress, Eucalyptus, Frankincense, Geranium,
Lavender, Patchouli, Rose, Sandalwood, Ylang Ylang

Sexual Problems

Sexual problems are best spoken about with a qualified physician, in order to rule out any underlying health concerns. A referral to a counsellor in order to have someone to talk to may also be helpful. However, in order to promote a relaxed yet gently stimulated mental state, try the balancing oils below.

Frigidity
How to use: Bath, inhalation, massage, skin oil, vaporisation.
Clary sage (postpartum), Jasmine (postpartum), Neroli, Patchouli, Sandalwood, Ylang Ylang.

Sexual overactivity
How to use: Bath, inhalation, massage, vaporisation.
Marjoram (postpartum)

Babies and Children

Between bumps and bruising, immunisations and bringing home every sniffle and splutter from play groups, children seem to be magnets for illness and disease. When your little one is under the weather, reach for a combination of the oils below. Again, please refer to "A Note on Oils for Babies and Children" for specific information, remember to only use a 1%, or one drop per teaspoon, dilution of essential oils, always perform a patch test before using a new oil, and never apply them to your child's face.

Aches and Pains
How to use: Bath, compress, massage
Chamomile, Clary Sage, Eucalyptus, Lavender, Marjoram, Peppermint, Rosemary, Thyme, Vetiver.

Asthma
How to use: Inhalation, massage, vaporisation
Clary Sage, Cypress, Eucalyptus, Frankincense, Lavender, Lemon, Marjoram, Peppermint, Rose, Rosemary, Tea Tree, Thyme.

Bruises
How to use: Compress, skin oil
Geranium, Lavender, Marjoram, Thyme.

Chickenpox
How to use: Bath, compress, skin oil
Bergamot, Chamomile, Eucalyptus, Lavender, Tea Tree.

Colds and Flu
How to use: Bath, inhalation, massage, vaporisation
Bergamot, Cedarwood, Cypress, Eucalyptus, Frankincense, Ginger, Lemon, Mandarin, Marjoram, Peppermint, Rose, Rosemary, Sandalwood, Tea Tree, Thyme.

Colic
How to use: Massage
Bergamot, Chamomile, Clary Sage, Ginger, Lavender, Mandarin, Marjoram, Neroli, Peppermint, Rosemary, Ylang Ylang.

Constipation
How to use: Massage, skin oil
Ginger, Mandarin, Rosemary.

Coughs
How to use: Inhalation, massage, vaporisation
Cedarwood, Clary Sage, Eucalyptus, Ginger, Marjoram, Rose, Rosemary, Tea Tree.

Cradle Cap
How to use: Skin oil
Cedarwood, Geranium, Lemon, Sandalwood.

Croup
How to use: Diffusion, massage
Marjoram, Sandalwood, Thyme

Inconsolable Crying

How to use: Diffusion, massage
Cypress, Chamomile, Frankincense, Geranium, Lavender, Rose, Ylang Ylang

Cuts and Sores
How to use: Compress, skin oil
Chamomile, Eucalyptus, Geranium, Lavender, Lime, Tea Tree, Thyme, Vetiver.

Digestion
How to use: Massage
Lemon, Mandarin

Dry, Sensitive Skin
How to use: Bath, flower water, massage, skin oil at a 1% dilution- 1 drop per 1 tsp of base oil
Bergamot, Cedarwood, Chamomile, Frankincense, Geranium, Jasmine, Lavender, Patchouli, Rose, Rosemary, Sandalwood, Thyme.

Earache
How to use: Compress made with good quality olive oil
Chamomile, Lavender, Tea Tree, Thyme

Fever
How to use: Bath, compress, diffusion
Bergamot, Eucalyptus, Ginger, Lavender, Lemon, Peppermint, Rosemary, Tea Tree, Thyme.

Headlice
How to use: Hair care, skin oil

Eucalyptus, Geranium, Lavender, Rosemary, Tea Tree, Thyme.

Hiccoughs
How to use: Diffusion
Mandarin

Insomnia
How to use: Bath, massage, vaporisation
Chamomile, Lavender, Mandarin, Marjoram, Neroli, Petitgrain, Rose, Sandalwood, Thyme.

Jaundice
How to use: Massage, skin oil
Geranium, Lemon, Mandarin, Rosemary.

NB- please do not use Lemon or Mandarin in conjunction with light therapy

Measles
How to use: Bath, inhalation, skin oil, vaporisation
Bergamot, Eucalyptus, Lavender, Tea Tree.

Nappy Rash
How to use: Massage, skin oil
Chamomile, Lavender

Nausea and Vomiting
How to use: Massage, vaporisation
Chamomile, Ginger, Lavender, Peppermint, Rose, Sandalwood.

<u>Premature</u>
Since all babies, though especially premature babies, have very thin and sensitive skin, it is best to avoid the use of essential oils.However, to combat stress and fatigue on your part, it may be worthwhile to diffuse Chamomile, Lavender, or some other oil you find personally soothing.

<u>Rashes</u>
How to use: Bath, compress, flower water, massage, skin oil
Chamomile, Lavender, Rose, Sandalwood, Tea Tree.

<u>Sore Throat and Throat Infection</u>
How to use: Inhalation, vaporisation
Bergamot, Clary Sage, Eucalyptus, Geranium, Ginger, Lavender, Sandalwood, Tea Tree, Thyme.

<u>Sprains and Strains</u>
How to use: Compress
Chamomile, Eucalyptus, Ginger, Jasmine, Lavender, Marjoram, Rosemary, Thyme, Vetiver.

<u>Teething Pain and Toothache</u>
How to use: Compress, skin oil
Bergamot, Chamomile, Clary Sage, Cypress, Lemon, Mandarin, Marjoram, Peppermint, Thyme.

<u>Thrush</u>
How to use: Massage

Geranium, Lavender, Lemon, Tea Tree, Thyme.

<u>Tonsillitis</u>
How to use: Skin oil
Chamomile, Ginger, Lavender, Lemon, Tea Tree.

<u>Whooping Cough</u>
How to use: Inhalation, massage
Clary Sage, Lavender, Rosemary, Tea Tree.

The Benefits of Meditation

Women are naturally contemplative creatures, our minds racing with all manner of thoughts throughout the day, which led me to make sure I gave recommendations for Natural Womanhood oils' use in meditative practices. In fact, all the oils listed in Essentially Feminine were first distilled for use in meditative or religious practice, many centuries ago. The first thing I am always asked about the oils is, "Well, how do you think I should meditate?"

My answer is always the same- Anything you do with awareness is meditation. Whether you sit quietly and enjoy the sensations of breathing, or listen to music, or knit, sew, work in the garden, take a walk or clean the house. When you focus completely on one activity, you are meditating.

You don't have to sit rigidly straight-backed staring at a candle, serenely chanting "Om..." adorned in mala beads, or working a Zen garden, though these thoughts come to mind when you hear the word "meditation" for a reason!

Thoughts may creep into your head, but if you notice them then let them go, rather than following them, you will learn to let them pass you by when you meditate. Taking time out to sit and do nothing is one of the hardest, but most rewarding parts of the day.

Some people ask the difference between meditation and

ritual, and I tell them "Meditation is not always ritual, but ritual is almost always meditative". After all, a ritual is a list of steps, done in a specific order, waiting to be assigned a reason or meaning.

Personally, I feel the best way to meditate is the way you find easiest to work into your day, as often as you can. A few suggestions that I use are:

- While brushing your teeth, in a morning and at night.
- Walking through a particular doorway in your home/office.
- Getting into your car/Entering your home- I use this one by touching a particular stone on the wall outside my home, and leaving the cares of the day at the door. Simple, but I'm always smiling as I turn the keys.
- Taking the time to enjoy making yourself a hot drink.

Bibliography

I would like to thank the following sources for my
continued study and growth, and for being my reference
sources throughout this process for information I
needed to recall, and facts I have had to check:

http://www.aromaweb.com, *the definitive essential oil
knowledge hub online*
Natural Health magazine, *a UK-based print magazine
dedicated to all forms of natural and alternative health*

The Essential Aromatherapy Book, *Carole McGilvery
and Jimi Reed*, 1995

The Handbook of Alternative Healing, *Raje Airey and
Jessica Houdret*, 2011

The Illustrated Encyclopedia of Essential Oils, *Julia
Lawless*, 1995

www.ingramcontent.com/pod-product-compliance
Lightning Source LLC
Chambersburg PA
CBHW022346290526
45786CB00014B/2508